GANSER SYNDROME NUTRITION

A Comprehensive Guide To Harnessing
Nutrition Power, Management And Mental
Wellness

Dr. Holmgren Alfred

the entities mentioned unless explicitly stated otherwise.

The author and publisher disclaim any liability or responsibility for any loss, injury, or damage caused by the use of the material offered in this book; readers use the information at their own risk.

All dietary and nutritional recommendations in this book are based on general principles and may not be suitable for everyone. Individual dietary needs and health conditions vary, so readers should consult with a healthcare professional to determine the best dietary choices for their specific circumstances.

By reading this book, you recognize and agree to the conditions of the disclaimer.

Ganser Syndrome Nutrition: With Expert Guidance" is an invaluable resource that delves into the intricate relationship between nutrition and mental health, particularly focusing on the often-overlooked condition of Ganser Syndrome. The comprehensive guide begins by providing a thorough understanding of Ganser Syndrome, tracing its origins, diagnostic criteria, prevalence, and various subtypes. It sets the stage by elucidating the complex etiology and risk factors associated

This book's central theme is the profound impact of nutrition on mental well-being, which is elucidated in the section dedicated to the intricate interplay of the gut-brain axis and the emerging field of nutritional psychiatry.

Through meticulous exploration, readers gain insight into how micronutrients and macronutrients influence psychological health and overall functioning. From the role of vitamins and minerals in managing Ganser Syndrome to the significance

By emphasizing lifestyle factors and nutritional interventions, such as exercise, sleep, and St.

One of the most compelling aspects of this book is the inclusion of real-life case studies and success stories, which give readers a glimpse into the transformative power of tailored nutritional interventions.

Through personal testimonies and insights from healthcare professionals, the book inspires hope and emphasizes the importance of personalized care in navigating the complexities of Ganser Syndrome.

The book "Ganser Syndrome Nutrition: With Expert Guidance" is a valuable resource for anyone looking to improve the quality of life for those suffering from Ganser Syndrome. It is a timely compilation of current knowledge that also points to future directions and emerging research.

CHAPTER 1
UNDERSTANDING GANSER'S SYNDROME

Overview of the Ganser Syndrome:

Ganser Syndrome, also known as "prison psychosis," is a rare dissociative disorder characterized by the presence of nonsensical or approximate answers to questions, often accompanied by dissociative symptoms such as depersonalization, derealization, and fugue states. First described by Sigbert Ganser in 1898, the syndrome has garnered attention due to its perplexing nature and its association with various psychiatric and neurological conditions. Individuals with Ga

History & Background:

Sabert Ganser, a German psychiatrist, first identified and documented the peculiar symptoms observed in certain patients in the late nineteenth century. Initially labeled as "hysterical pseudodementia," the syndrome gained recognition as a distinct dissociative disorder over time. Early research primarily focused on case reports and clinical observations, shedding light on the syndrome's clinical presentation and differentiation.

Diagnostic criteria:

The diagnosis of Ganser Syndrome is based on specific criteria outlined in psychiatric classification systems, such as the DSM-5. According to the DSM-5, key features of Ganser Syndrome are the presence of approximate answers to questions, dissociative symptoms, and a lack of intention to deceive. These symptoms must occur in the absence of severe cognitive impairment or another underlying psychiatric condition. Clinicians typically rely on structured clinical interviews.

Ganser Syndrome is considered extremely rare, with limited epidemiological data available regarding its prevalence and incidence rates. Because of its elusive nature and diagnostic challenges, accurately estimating the prevalence of Ganser Syndrome poses significant difficulties.

The syndrome is believed to occur more frequently in certain populations, such as incarcerated individuals or those with a history of severe trauma or stress.

Subtypes And Variants:

While Ganser Syndrome is recognized as a distinct clinical entity, it may manifest in various subtypes or variants, each characterized by unique clinical features and presentations.

Variants of Ganser Syndrome may coexist with other psychiatric conditions, such as mood disorders, personality disorders, or substance use disorders.

Etiology And Risk Factors:

Ganser Syndrome's etiology is multifactorial and poorly understood, with no single cause identified to account for its development. Several potential etiological factors and risk markers have been proposed based on clinical observations and theoretical models, including psychosocial stressors, traumatic experiences, underlying psychiatric conditions, neurobiological abnormalities, and genetics.

CHAPTER 2
NUTRITION'S IMPACT ON MENTAL HEALTH

Research in the field of nutritional psychiatry has highlighted the intricate relationship between dietary patterns and mental health outcomes. Poor dietary choices, characterized by the consumption of processed foods high in sugar, saturated fats, and refined carbohydrates, have been linked.

The Gut-Brain Axis:

Dysbiosis, or imbalances in gut microbiota composition, has been linked to the pathogenesis of various diseases. The gut-brain axis is a bidirectional communication pathway that connects the gastrointestinal tract and the central nervous system, encompassing neural, hormonal, and immunological signaling mechanisms.

Nutritional Psychiatry Overview And Concepts:

Nutritional psychiatry is an interdisciplinary field that investigates the relationship between diet, nutrients, and mental health outcomes. It encompasses the study of how dietary factors influence brain function, neurotransmitter synthesis, neuroinflammation, and synaptic plasticity, eventually shaping mood, cognition, and behavior. Nutritional psychiatry takes a holistic approach to mental health care, emphasizing the importance of dietary interventions as adjunctive or

Micronutrients And Mental Health:

Micronutrients, including vitamins, minerals, and trace elements, play essential roles in neurodevelopment, neurotransmitter synthesis, and neuronal signaling pathways implicated in mental health. Deficiencies in key micronutrients such as folate, vitamin B12, vitamin D, iron, zinc, and magnesium have been linked to an increased risk of depression, anxiety, and cognitive impairment. Supplementation with micronutrients, either as monotherapy or adjunctive therapy,

Macronutrients And Mental Health:

Macronutrients, which include carbohydrates, proteins, and fats, provide energy to the body and serve as building blocks for cellular structures, neurotransmitters, and hormones involved in brain function and mental health regulation. The quality and composition of macronutrient intake influence neurotransmitter synthesis, neuroinflammation, oxidative stress, and synaptic plasticity, thereby impacting mood, cognition, and emotional resilience. High-quality carbohydrates,

Dietary patterns, defined by the overall composition, variety, and frequency of food consumption, exert profound effects on psychological well-being and mental health outcomes. Traditional dietary patterns, such as the Mediterranean diet and the DASH diet, characterized by an abundance of fruits, vegetables, whole grains, nuts, seeds, and lean proteins, have been associated with a lower risk of depression, anxiety, and cognitive

CHAPTER 3
NUTRITIONAL CONSIDERATIONS FOR GANSER SYNDROME

Ganser Syndrome, a rare dissociative disorder characterized by the presence of approximate answers, confusion, and clouded consciousness, poses significant challenges for those affected and their caregivers. While the primary focus of treatment is typically psychotherapy and pharmacotherapy, the role of nutrition in managing Ganser Syndrome should not be overlooked. Nutritional considerations play a vital role in the holistic approach to treating individuals.

Nutritional Implications For Ganser Syndrome Management

Adequate nutrient intake is essential for maintaining optimal brain function and supporting neurotransmitter balance, which are crucial factors in managing the symptoms associated with Ganser Syndrome. Certain nutrients, such as vitamins B6, B12, and folate, play key roles in neurotransmitter synthesis and function, and deficiencies in these nutrients have been linked to a variety of mental health disorders.

A diet rich in antioxidants, omega-3 fatty acids, and other micronutrients has been linked to improved mood, cognitive performance, and overall mental health.

On the other hand, a diet high in processed foods, sugar, and unhealthy fats may exacerbate symptoms and contribute to worsened mental functioning, so diet

Individuals with Ganser Syndrome frequently suffer from nutritional deficiencies, which can exacerbate symptoms and impair overall well-being. These deficiencies can be caused by a variety of factors, including poor dietary habits, malabsorption issues, medication side effects, and increased nutrient demands due to stress or illness.

Vitamin B12 deficiency, in particular, is common and is associated with cognitive impairment, mood disturbances, and

Individuals with Ganser Syndrome may also have deficiencies in other essential nutrients, such as folate, vitamin B6, zinc, and magnesium. These nutrients play critical roles in neurotransmitter synthesis, DNA methylation, and antioxidant defense mechanisms, all of which are implicated in mental health and cognitive function. Addressing these deficiencies through dietary changes and targeted supplementation is essential for optimizing

Dietary Factors Associated with Ganser Syndrome Symptoms

Excessive consumption of caffeine, alcohol, and sugar has been linked to increased anxiety, irritability, and cognitive dysfunction, all of which can worsen the symptoms of Ganser Syndrome. Dietary factors can also have a significant impact on the severity and frequency of symptoms.

Moreover, processed foods high in refined carbohydrates, unhealthy fats, and artificial additives may contribute to inflammation and oxidative stress in the brain, further exacerbating psychiatric symptoms. On the other hand, a diet rich in whole foods, including fruits, vegetables, whole grains, lean proteins, and healthy fats, provides essential nutrients and antioxidants that support optimal brain function and mental well-being. Thus, adopting a nutrient-dense diet

Nutritional Support Strategies

Nutritional support strategies encompass a range of interventions aimed at addressing specific nutrient deficiencies, improving overall health, and optimizing mental well-being in individuals with Ganser Syndrome. These strategies may include dietary modifications, supplementation, and lifestyle interventions designed to support optimal nutrition and improve treatment outcomes.

To begin, dietary interventions should promote a well-balanced eating pattern that emphasizes nutrient-dense foods while minimizing processed and unhealthy options. This could entail collaborating with a registered dietitian or nutritionist to create personalized meal plans tailored to individual needs and preferences.

In addition to dietary changes, targeted supplementation may be required to address specific nutrient deficiencies identified through blood tests or clinical assessment. Supplementation with vitamins B12, B6, and folate, as well as other key nutrients such as zinc, magnesium, and omega-3 fatty acids, may be beneficial in supporting mental health and cognitive function in individuals with Ganser Syndrome.

Furthermore, prioritizing adequate sleep, stress management techniques and regular exercise are integral components of holistic nutritional support for Ganser Syndrome.

Physical activity has been shown to improve mood, reduce anxiety, and enhance cognitive function, while stress management techniques like mindfulness meditation and deep breathing exercises can help regulate emotions and promote mental well-being.

nutritional considerations play a crucial role in the management of Ganser Syndrome. Addressing nutrient deficiencies, optimizing dietary intake, and implementing lifestyle interventions can complement traditional treatment modalities and improve overall outcomes for individuals with this disorder. Healthcare providers can help empower individuals with Ganser Syndrome by taking a holistic approach to nutrition and mental health.

CHAPTER 4
MICRONUTRIENTS AND GANSER'S SYNDROME

Micronutrients play a crucial role in the maintenance of overall health and well-being, including mental health. In the context of Ganser Syndrome, a rare dissociative disorder characterized by the presence of nonsensical or approximate answers to questions, understanding the impact of micronutrients becomes paramount. Vitamin deficiencies have been implicated in various mental health disorders, and Ganser Syndrome is no exception. Deficiencies in certain vitamins, such as B vitamins (particularly B12 and folate), vitamin D, and vitamin E, have been associated with cognitive dysfunction, mood disturbances, and neurological symptoms, all of which are relevant to the manifestation of Ganser Syndrome.

For instance, B12 deficiency can lead to cognitive impairment, memory deficits, and confusion, which may exacerbate the symptoms of Ganser Syndrome.

Similarly, inadequate levels of vitamin D have been linked to depression and cognitive decline, potentially worsening the condition in individuals with Ganser Syndrome. Therefore, ensuring adequate intake of these vitamins through diet and supplementation may be beneficial in managing symptoms and promoting mental wellness in individuals with Ganser Syndrome.

In addition to vitamins, mineral deficiencies can also contribute to the development and exacerbation of Ganser Syndrome. Minerals such as iron, zinc, magnesium, and selenium are essential for proper brain function and mood regulation, and deficiencies in these minerals have been linked to cognitive dysfunction, mood disorders, and altered neurotransmitter activity, all of which are relevant to the pathophysiology of Ganser Syndrome.

Micronutrient supplementation represents a potential therapeutic approach for individuals with Ganser Syndrome, particularly those with identified deficiencies. While obtaining essential nutrients through a balanced diet is ideal, supplementation may be necessary to address existing deficiencies and support optimal mental health. However, it is essential to approach supplementation cautiously and under the guidance of a healthcare professional, as excessive intake of certain micronutrients can have adverse effects and may interact with medications commonly prescribed for Ganser Syndrome. Moreover, individual variability in nutrient absorption and metabolism should be taken into account when determining the appropriate dosage and formulation of supplements. Additionally, supplementation should complement rather than replace dietary intake, emphasizing the importance of consuming a varied and nutrient-rich diet. Overall, micronutrient supplementation may serve as a valuable adjunctive therapy in the management of Ganser Syndrome, but careful consideration of individual needs and potential risks is essential to ensure its efficacy and safety.

CHAPTER 5
MACRONUTRIENTS AND GANSER'S SYNDROME

Understanding the impact of macronutrients on mental health and cognition is crucial in managing Ganser Syndrome, a rare dissociative disorder characterized by the presence of pseudo-intellectual responses, confusion, and perceptual disturbances. Carbohydrates, proteins, and fats are the three primary macronutrients that provide the body with energy and essential nutrients required for its proper functioning.

Carbohydrates are the body's primary source of energy, especially for the brain. They are broken down into glucose, which fuels neuronal activity and supports cognitive functions such as memory, attention, and decision-making.

However, the type and quality of carbohydrates consumed can significantly influence mental wellness. Complex carbohydrates found in whole grains, fruits, and vegetables provide sustained energy release and promote stable blood sugar levels.

Consuming adequate protein sources, such as lean meats, fish, eggs, dairy products, legumes, and nuts, can help balance neurotransmitters, which are chemical messengers that facilitate communication between neurons in the brain. Amino acids, the building blocks of proteins, play an important role in neurotransmitter production, including serotonin and dopamine, which are implicated in mood regulation and cognitive function.

Adequate intake of healthy fats is essential for optimizing neurotransmitter function, promoting

Balanced macronutrient intake is essential for individuals with Ganser Syndrome to support overall health and well-being. A diet that incorporates a variety of nutrient-dense foods from all three macronutrient groups can help stabilize mood, improve cognitive function, and enhance overall mental wellness. Moreover, maintaining balanced blood sugar levels through the consumption of complex carbohydrates, lean proteins, and healthy fats can help prevent energy crashes and mood fluctuations commonly experienced by individuals with Ganser Syndrome. Working with a qualified healthcare professional or registered dietitian to develop a personalized nutrition plan tailored to individual needs and preferences is recommended for optimal management of Ganser Syndrome. Additionally, integrating lifestyle modifications such as regular physical activity, stress management techniques, and adequate sleep can complement dietary interventions and promote holistic wellness in individuals living with Ganser Syndrome.

CHAPTER 6
DIETARY PATTERNS AND GANSER'S SYNDROME

Dietary patterns encompass the overall composition and variety of foods consumed, which can significantly influence physical health and mental well-being.

Research suggests that certain dietary patterns may either exacerbate or alleviate symptoms associated with Ganser Syndrome.

Mediterranean Diet with Ganser Syndrome:

The Mediterranean diet has garnered significant attention for its potential benefits in promoting overall health and well-being, including mental health. Characterized by a high consumption of fruits, vegetables, whole grains, legumes, nuts, and olive oil, along with a moderate intake of fish, poultry, and dairy, the Mediterranean diet offers a rich source of essential nutrients, antioxidants, and healthy fats. Studies have indicated that adherence to the Mediterranean diet may be associated with reduced risk of depression and cognitive decline, both of which are pertinent to individuals with Ganser Syndrome.

The anti-inflammatory properties of this diet, attributed to its abundance of omega-3 fatty acids and phytochemicals, may also contribute to mitigating neuroinflammation, which has been implicated in various psychiatric disorders, including Ganser Syndrome. Additionally, the Mediterranean diet's emphasis on whole foods and nutrient-dense ingredients aligns with the principles of holistic nutrition, supporting overall mental wellness and cognitive function in individuals affected by Ganser Syndrome.

DASH Diet With Ganser Syndrome:

The Dietary Approaches to Stop Hypertension (DASH) diet is another dietary pattern that has been extensively studied for its health benefits, particularly in managing cardiovascular health and reducing hypertension. The DASH diet prioritizes the consumption of fruits, vegetables, whole grains, lean proteins, and low-fat dairy products while limiting sodium, saturated fats, and refined sugars. While its primary focus is on cardiovascular health, the DASH diet's emphasis on nutrient-rich foods and balanced nutrition can also positively impact mental health outcomes, potentially benefiting individuals with Ganser Syndrome. By promoting cardiovascular health and improving blood flow to the brain, the DASH diet may enhance cognitive function and mood regulation, thereby complementing therapeutic interventions for Ganser Syndrome. Moreover, the DASH diet's emphasis on sodium restriction may be particularly relevant, as excessive salt intake has been linked to cognitive impairment and psychiatric symptoms, which individuals with Ganser Syndrome may be susceptible to.

Plant-Based Diets And The Ganser Syndrome:

Plant-based diets, characterized by the predominance of fruits, vegetables, grains, nuts, seeds, and legumes while excluding or minimizing animal products, have gained popularity for their potential health benefits and sustainability. Numerous studies have associated plant-based diets with reduced risk of chronic diseases, including cardiovascular disease, diabetes, and certain cancers.

 In the context of Ganser Syndrome, adopting a plant-based diet may offer several advantages. Firstly, plant-based diets are rich in fiber, vitamins, minerals, and phytonutrients, which support overall health and immune function, potentially reducing the risk of inflammation and oxidative stress associated with psychiatric disorders. Secondly, plant-based diets are typically lower in saturated fats and cholesterol, which have been implicated in cognitive decline and mood disorders.

By promoting cardiovascular health and metabolic balance, plant-based diets may indirectly support mental wellness in individuals with Ganser Syndrome. Additionally, the ethical and environmental considerations inherent in plant-based diets may contribute to improved psychological well-being and sense of connectedness, factors that are relevant to holistic approaches in managing Ganser Syndrome.

Keto Diet And Ganser Syndrome:

The ketogenic diet, characterized by high fat, moderate protein, and very low carbohydrate intake, has gained attention for its therapeutic potential in various neurological and psychiatric disorders.

By inducing a state of ketosis, wherein the body utilizes ketones as an alternative fuel source, the ketogenic diet has been shown to modulate neurotransmitter function, reduce inflammation, and enhance mitochondrial function, all of which may be relevant to individuals with Ganser Syndrome. While research specifically examining the ketogenic diet in Ganser Syndrome is limited, studies in related conditions such as epilepsy and mood disorders have demonstrated promising results.

The neuroprotective effects of ketones, particularly beta-hydroxybutyrate (BHB), may mitigate neuronal dysfunction and excitotoxicity, potentially improving cognitive function and mood regulation in individuals with Ganser Syndrome. Moreover, the ketogenic diet's ability to stabilize blood sugar levels and regulate energy metabolism may contribute to enhanced mental clarity and emotional stability, factors that are pertinent to managing Ganser Syndrome symptoms. However, it is essential to consider individual variability and potential side effects of the ketogenic diet, such as electrolyte imbalances and gastrointestinal issues, when implementing this dietary approach for Ganser Syndrome management.

Further research is warranted to elucidate the efficacy and safety of the ketogenic diet in this population, particularly in conjunction with standard treatments and holistic interventions.

CHAPTER 7

LIFESTYLE FACTORS AND NUTRITIONAL INTERVENTIONS

The management of Ganser Syndrome necessitates a comprehensive approach that extends beyond conventional medical treatments. Lifestyle factors, particularly nutrition, play a crucial role in influencing the course of the syndrome and overall mental wellness.

Exercise And Ganser Syndrome

Regular physical exercise has emerged as a fundamental aspect of managing Ganser Syndrome. Engaging in structured exercise routines can yield numerous benefits for individuals dealing with this condition. Physical activity stimulates the release of endorphins, neurotransmitters known for their mood-enhancing properties, thereby potentially alleviating symptoms of depression and anxiety that commonly co-occur with Ganser Syndrome. Furthermore, exercise promotes neuroplastic

Individuals with Ganser Syndrome frequently experience sleep disturbances, which exacerbate their cognitive dysfunction and emotional instability. To manage this aspect of the syndrome, it is critical to prioritize adequate sleep hygiene.

Creating a sleep-friendly environment, sticking to a regular sleep schedule, and practicing relaxation techniques before bedtime can help regulate sleep patterns and improve sleep quality. Additionally, dietary changes, such as limiting

Stress Management and the Ganser Syndrome

Mindfulness meditation, deep breathing exercises, and progressive muscle relaxation are some of the techniques that can modulate the body's stress response and promote emotional resilience in people with Ganser Syndrome. Because stress has a significant impact on the manifestation and exacerbation of Ganser Syndrome symptoms, it is critical to implement effective stress management strategies to optimize treatment outcomes.

Behavioral Interventions To Improve Nutrition.

Cognitive-behavioral therapy (CBT), for example, can help individuals identify and challenge maladaptive thoughts and behaviors related to food and body image, fostering a more

lifestyle factors and nutritional interventions constitute integral components of the multifaceted approach to managing Ganser Syndrome. By addressing factors such as exercise, sleep, stress, and dietary behaviors, healthcare professionals can optimize treatment outcomes and enhance the quality of life for individuals dealing with this complex disorder. Implementing evidence-based strategies tailored to each individual's unique needs is essential in

CHAPTER 8
PRACTICAL TIPS FOR MANAGING NUTRITION IN GANSER'S SYNDROME

Nutrition plays a crucial role in managing any mental health disorder, including Ganser Syndrome, as it can affect mood stability, cognitive function, and overall well-being. As a rare dissociative disorder characterized by symptomatology such as approximate answers, clouding of consciousness, and dissociative amnesia, Ganser Syndrome presents unique challenges in effectively managing nutrition.

Meal Planning and Preparation Strategies

Creating a weekly or monthly meal plan that takes into account dietary preferences, nutritional needs, and budget constraints is an important part of ensuring that people with Ganser Syndrome eat a well-balanced and nutritious diet. Planning meals ahead of time allows for the incorporation of nutrient-dense foods that are necessary for brain health and cognitive function. Meal preparation strategies include

Grocery Shopping For Nutritional Success

Creating a detailed shopping list based on a predetermined meal plan can help streamline the shopping process and prevent impulse purchases of unhealthy items. This is especially important for people with Ganser Syndrome, who may struggle with concentration and decision-making. Prioritizing whole foods like fruits and vegetables

Dining Out And Social Situations

Participating in social gatherings and dining out at restaurants are common activities that may present challenges for individuals with Ganser Syndrome in maintaining optimal nutrition. However, with careful planning and preparation, it is possible to navigate these situations while prioritizing mental wellness. Before dining out, researching restaurant menus in advance can help identify healthier options and accommodate any dietary restrictions or preferences. Communicating openly with friends or dining companions about specific dietary needs can also alleviate feelings of discomfort or embarrassment. Additionally, practicing mindful eating techniques, such as slowing down the pace of eating and paying attention to hunger cues, can enhance the dining experience and promote satiety. By proactively addressing potential triggers or stressors associated with social eating occasions, individuals with Ganser Syndrome can cultivate a positive relationship with food and foster mental well-being.

Overcoming Obstacles To Healthy Eating

Various barriers may hinder individuals with Ganser Syndrome from maintaining a consistent and nutritious diet.

These barriers can range from cognitive impairments and executive functioning deficits to socio-economic constraints and environmental influences.

Therefore, it is crucial to identify and address these barriers effectively to facilitate adherence to healthy eating habits. Utilizing cognitive-behavioral strategies, such as cognitive restructuring and problem-solving techniques, can help individuals with Ganser Syndrome overcome cognitive distortions and make informed food choices. Seeking support from mental health professionals, dietitians, or support groups can provide valuable guidance and encouragement in navigating nutritional challenges. Moreover, addressing socio-economic barriers through community resources, such as food assistance programs or affordable meal delivery services, can ensure access to nutritious foods regardless of financial constraints.

By implementing personalized strategies tailored to individual needs and circumstances, individuals with Ganser Syndrome can overcome barriers to healthy eating and optimize their nutritional intake for improved mental wellness.

managing nutrition effectively is essential for individuals with Ganser Syndrome to support their mental health and overall well-being. By implementing practical strategies such as meal planning and preparation, navigating grocery shopping and dining out, and overcoming barriers to healthy eating, individuals with Ganser Syndrome can cultivate a positive relationship with food and enhance their quality of life. Collaborating with healthcare professionals,

CHAPTER 9
CASE STUDIES AND SUCCESS STORIES

In the realm of Ganser Syndrome management, case studies and success stories serve as invaluable resources for understanding the efficacy of nutritional interventions. These accounts provide detailed narratives of individuals who have undergone specific dietary changes or implemented nutritional strategies to alleviate symptoms associated with Ganser Syndrome. By examining these cases, researchers and healthcare professionals can glean insights into the diverse ways in which nutrition impacts mental wellness in individuals with this disorder. Case studies offer a comprehensive view of the holistic approach to treatment, shedding light on the interplay between diet, psychological factors, and symptomatology. Moreover, they highlight the importance of personalized dietary interventions tailored to the unique needs of each individual, emphasizing the significance of a multidisciplinary approach in Ganser Syndrome management. Success stories not only inspire hope but also underscore the potential for meaningful improvements in mental health outcomes through targeted nutritional interventions. These narratives provide anecdotal evidence of the transformative power of nutrition in enhancing the well-being and quality of life of individuals grappling with Ganser Syndrome. By analyzing the factors contributing to successful outcomes, such as adherence to dietary recommendations, lifestyle modifications, and ongoing support from healthcare professionals, stakeholders can glean valuable insights into best practices for integrating nutrition into comprehensive treatment plans for Ganser Syndrome.

Real-world Examples of Nutritional Interventions:

Real-life examples of nutritional interventions offer tangible evidence of the impact of dietary modifications on symptom management and mental wellness in individuals with Ganser Syndrome.

These examples encompass a wide range of dietary approaches, including supplementation with specific nutrients, adoption of therapeutic diets, and elimination of potential trigger foods.

By examining the outcomes of these interventions, researchers and practitioners can elucidate the mechanisms underlying the relationship between nutrition and

Ganser Syndrome, thereby informing evidence-based treatment protocols. Additionally, real-life examples provide valuable insights into the practical challenges and barriers associated with implementing dietary changes in clinical settings and everyday life.

Through detailed documentation of dietary protocols, adherence strategies, and monitoring mechanisms, these examples contribute to the development of tailored nutritional interventions that optimize outcomes for individuals with Ganser Syndrome. Furthermore, they underscore the importance of ongoing evaluation and adjustment of dietary regimens based on individual responses and evolving clinical needs. By sharing their experiences and outcomes, individuals who have undergone nutritional interventions for Ganser Syndrome play a crucial role in advancing understanding and awareness of the role of nutrition in mental health management.

Personal testimonies from individuals with Ganser Syndrome offer firsthand accounts of the challenges, experiences, and triumphs associated with navigating the complexities of this disorder.

These testimonies provide unique insights into the lived experiences of individuals grappling with Ganser Syndrome, shedding light on the multifaceted nature of their journey toward recovery and resilience. Through sharing their stories, individuals with Ganser Syndrome not only raise awareness about the disorder but also provide valuable perspectives on the role of nutrition in their healing process. Personal testimonies often highlight the pivotal role of dietary interventions in symptom management and overall well-being, offering hope and encouragement to others facing similar challenges. Moreover, these testimonies foster a sense of community and solidarity among individuals with Ganser Syndrome, creating a supportive environment for sharing coping strategies, resources, and insights into effective self-care practices. By amplifying the voices of those directly affected by the disorder, personal testimonies contribute to destigmatizing mental health conditions and advocating for holistic approaches to treatment that prioritize the integration of nutrition and other lifestyle factors.

Perspectives From Healthcare Professionals:

Insights from healthcare professionals are essential for synthesizing empirical evidence, clinical expertise, and patient perspectives to inform comprehensive approaches to Ganser Syndrome management. Healthcare professionals, including psychiatrists, dietitians, psychologists, and other allied health professionals, play a central role in assessing, diagnosing, and treating individuals with Ganser Syndrome.

Their insights encompass a broad spectrum of knowledge, ranging from the neurobiological basis of the disorder to the practical considerations involved in implementing nutritional interventions within clinical practice.

Healthcare professionals offer critical perspectives on the evidence base supporting the role of nutrition in mental health, elucidating the mechanisms through which dietary factors influence symptomatology and treatment outcomes in Ganser Syndrome.

Additionally, they guide the development and implementation of personalized nutrition plans tailored to the unique needs and preferences of individuals with Ganser Syndrome. By collaborating with other members of the healthcare team and engaging in interdisciplinary dialogue, healthcare professionals facilitate holistic and integrated approaches to Ganser Syndrome management that prioritize the optimization of nutritional status alongside pharmacological and psychosocial interventions. Through ongoing research, education, and advocacy efforts, healthcare professionals contribute to advancing the field of nutritional psychiatry and promoting the integration of nutrition into mainstream mental healthcare paradigms.

CHAPTER 10
FUTURE DIRECTIONS AND CONCLUSIONS

Emerging Research in Nutrition and the Ganser Syndrome

The exploration of nutrition's impact on Ganser Syndrome represents a burgeoning field in mental health research. Despite limited current literature specifically addressing the intersection of nutrition and Ganser Syndrome, emerging studies suggest promising avenues for further investigation. Recent research has underscored the role of certain nutrients, such as omega-3 fatty acids, B vitamins, and antioxidants, in supporting cognitive function and mental well-being, which may have implications for individuals with Ganser Syndrome. Additionally, investigations into the gut-brain axis have highlighted the potential influence of gut health and microbiota composition on mental health disorders, including those characterized by cognitive disturbances like Ganser Syndrome. Future research endeavors could delve deeper into elucidating the mechanisms underlying the relationship between nutrition and Ganser Syndrome, potentially uncovering novel therapeutic strategies or preventive measures. Furthermore, longitudinal studies assessing the efficacy of dietary interventions and nutritional supplementation in managing Ganser Syndrome symptoms are warranted to provide evidence-based recommendations for clinical practice.

Challenges and Opportunities

Navigating the landscape of nutrition and Ganser Syndrome research presents several challenges and opportunities.

One significant challenge is the inherent complexity and heterogeneity of Ganser Syndrome itself, which may complicate efforts to identify specific dietary patterns or nutritional interventions that are universally beneficial. Additionally, methodological limitations, such as small sample sizes and lack of rigorous study designs, pose obstacles to generating robust evidence in this area. Moreover, addressing confounding variables, such as comorbidities and medication use, is essential to elucidate the true relationship between nutrition and Ganser Syndrome. Despite these challenges, there are several opportunities for advancement. Collaborative interdisciplinary research efforts involving nutritionists, psychiatrists, neuroscientists, and other relevant disciplines can foster a comprehensive understanding of the multifaceted interactions between diet and mental health in Ganser Syndrome. Utilizing advanced analytical techniques, such as metabolomics and microbiome profiling, may offer insights into the metabolic and microbial signatures associated with Ganser Syndrome, potentially informing personalized nutritional interventions. Moreover, leveraging digital health technologies, such as mobile apps and wearable devices, can facilitate real-time monitoring of dietary intake and symptomatology, enhancing both research methodologies and clinical management strategies.

FINAL THOUGHTS

In conclusion, while the field of nutrition and Ganser Syndrome is still in its infancy, recent advances in research provide optimism for the potential role of nutrition in managing this enigmatic disorder. Moving forward, it is imperative to prioritize rigorous scientific inquiry to elucidate the complex interplay between diet, gut health, and cognitive function in Ganser Syndrome. Clinicians should consider incorporating dietary assessment and nutritional counseling into the comprehensive management of individuals with Ganser Syndrome, recognizing the potential impact of dietary factors on symptom severity and overall well-being. Additionally, public health initiatives aimed at promoting healthy dietary habits and optimizing nutritional status may have broader implications for reducing the burden of mental health disorders, including Ganser Syndrome, at the population level.

Ultimately, by embracing a holistic approach that integrates nutritional considerations into the care continuum, we can strive towards improving outcomes and enhancing the quality of life for individuals affected by Ganser Syndrome.